thomas propp

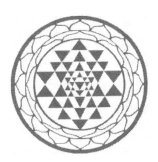

meridian-stretching
partner yoga practice

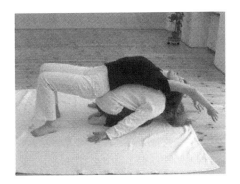

berlin 2009
www.yogalila.de

0

contents

meridian-stretching partner yoga practice
thomas propp
english translation by julie blumenthal
copyright: © 2012 thomas propp

1. introduction

for around the past two years, i have been integrating one or more meridian-stretching partner exercises into my yoga classes. i was encouraged in this by a seminar with daniel orlansky in bad sulza in 2007, as well as previous and parallel experiences with various forms of body work, primarily shiatsu, traditional thai massage and aikido.

contact with a partner is not an original element of hatha-yoga. through yoga practice, one comes to sense one's own energies, either through the instructions or examples of a teacher, or by being gently guided or brought into them by a knowing hand. true yoga is meant to be experienced in self study, in sustained quiet effort done for oneself. useful poses are learned in group class, and then practiced at home.

why then open up this original, individual yoga practice to partner contact?

the answer to this is: because it can facilitate and enhance the possibilities of yoga. brand-new beginners often find it difficult to experience intensity in a pose. partner work can facilitate this. the partner can give stability and security; optimally, one can then more easily and completely surrender, and thereby more completely experience the beauty of the inner solution.

i was trained in hatha-yoga, which stems from tantric traditions. this means all the senses are specifically directed in the endeavour of awakening the body from its self-inflicted sleep. thus the work is not leading to something like health or suppleness, or increased age or even enlightenment; rather the goal of the effort is the removal of goals, in view of freedom.

only in this way is life reordered, the body made strong, the breath schooled, the spirit directed and refined; so that the yoga practice can more and more completely, more and more often, tear through the fog of everyday perceptions and arrive in clear sight of the happiness of existence. this is a movement towards beauty. the present is experienced just as it is, and because the experience is so complete, one's inner beauty comes to the fore. experience, which seizes on every nuance and facet of a part of the world, trembles before its beauty.

this happens through the intense practice of yoga, and particularly easily in the exchange with a fellow human who touches you.

this is what i want to present with this work.

thomas propp
berlin, august 2009

2. nadis and meridians, presentation and comparison of concepts

yoga exercises are easily distinguished from each other with respect to their direction of movement: forward bends, backbends, side bends, twists, inversions. thereby different areas of the body are challenged and stretched. this external description can be set against a contemplation of the inner experience, which concerns itself with the energy flow of the body.

the indian side of the world

according to indian doctrine, the kundalini serpent, coiled three and a half times, sits at the first chakra (muladhara, the pelvic floor). kundalini is the power of shakti, the creative aspect of shiva, the lord of the world. shakti is mythologically referred to as the consort of shiva. shakti's kundalini force (kundalini shakti) creates all of life. in everyday life, she wants to stay quiet, asleep at the pelvic floor. when the kundalini sleeps, our awareness of the illusions of the world is trapped. through yoga or other providential occurrences, kundalini can come into motion, and slowly or quickly find the way up, back from where she came: back to shiva, lord of all, to an unfettered view of the world. her path travels the primary energy meridian, susumna nadi in the spinal cord, up to the seventh chakra and beyond. the phenomena that are reported from this travel will not be discussed here; in any case, it is a way out of inhibition, out of our energetic bonds, to freedom.

the yogic sources describe, neighboring susumna nadi, a network of main and secondary nadis. it has been counted as 300,000, then again as 200,000 or 72,000 or even fourteen, but in general, 10 are known. target points appear: nostril, eye, ear, mouth, the genitals, but also the anus and heels. in any case the ida (moon) and pingala (sun) nadis entwine susumna, the central nadi. mircea eliade, from whom i have taken this information, writes in his book *yoga - immortality and freedom* on page 248: "the texts repeat insistently that in the uninitiated, the nadi becomes 'unclean', is 'clogged' must be 'cleansed' through the practice of asana, pranayama and mudra (reference, for example, HY-Pr. i.58) "

japan's chinese contribution

around 100 years ago, chinese medicine, with its doctrine of energy meridians, came to japan. there, a culture of "finger pressure" (shiatsu) massage, based on the meridians, developed. in the end, shitsuto masunaga broke away from the form of acupuncture and used these principles to work directly with the meridians on the body.

in the 1970s, masunaga himself called his art *zen-shiatsu* and described that in a meditative, clairvoyant state, he could actually "see" the meridians. the traditional concept, in which the meridians were organized around the organs or „elemental phases of transformation", was then adopted from him and expanded.

wilfried rappenecker, a well-known german shiatsu teacher, writes, "we can understand the flow in the meridians as the expression of the flow of the universal life energy within us. unimpeded flow here means spiritual, mental and physical wellbeing, stable movement and progression. disabilities arise when we close off a portion of our body and soul from the flow of the universal life force. what follows in these sites is stagnation of our further development at all levels ... "(rappenecker, wilfried, *shiatsu for beginners*, p. 11)

an experienced shiatsu practitioner can work therapeutically, through a diagnosis of the energy conditions in the five elemental phases. in contrast, in the context of a yoga class meridian stretching has a balancing and cleansing effect on them. rappenecker emphasizes the meditative effect on both parties, the giving and the receiving partner. he speaks of a "non-intentional communication" (op. cit., p.13)

shiatsu is based on 14 meridians, of which 12 are divided into a cycle of five elemental phases of transformation: fire, earth, metal, water, wood, joining in two of the primary meridians, the „conception vessel" and the „governing vessel".

the first 12 meridians are associated with specific organs: lung, large intestine, stomach, spleen, heart, small intestine, bladder, kidney, pericardium, triple warmer (an imagined, "new" organ), gallbladder and liver. it is understood in shiatsu that the organ does not reference the physical organ, but rather the energetic representative site in the overall microstructure of the energetic-somatic organism. the lung is for example the quality of communication, the large intestine the quality of release, the kidney the quality of vitality or inherited universal life energy, and so on. this is mentioned here only to explain and illustrate the environment in which meridian work takes place. this knowledge is not required for the practice of meridian stretching exercises in yoga. in continuing developments of many of the classic shiatsu practices, for example in the hara-awareness massage of ananda würzburg, the context of the meridians is not necessary to the successful work of the practitioner.

during shiatsu, pressure is applied not only with fingers but also with other body parts: elbow, knee, fist. this pressure is also not only pushed, but pulled! it is important that this work is not a push or a pull in isolation; rather every movement should be led from the center of the body outward; the keyword here is "lean" rather than press or push. body weight is applied in as comfortable and tension-free a way as possible. thus, the relaxed bearing of the practitioner or active partner transfers to their receiving partner.

india, china, japan...

we can state with certainty that eastern body considerations arise from a system of energy lines, whose sensible treatment corrects energy imbalances and brings blockages back into flow.

3. psycho-dynamic aspects of partner and group exercises in yoga teaching

not every man or woman enjoys being touched by another. all experiences of touch and being touched can be present at once, when your yoga partner places their hand or foot or knee on you. different cultures respond differently to physical contact; individuals may carry minor or even major traumas with them, as part of their life story.

also, the active contact may itself be problematic. certainly, maybe i enjoy touching my romantic partner. but just anyone? perhaps it transmits illness? perhaps i just do not like his or her energy enough that i want to meet him or her skin to skin? i have simply never touched a stranger this way: who knows what could happen?

all these questions affect partner practice in yoga, and can create problems within it. i once experienced a participant who said they did not like it, and didn't return. another - of perhaps 200 students - expressed, they would prefer it if i did not teach partner exercises *so often*. from the others, i continuously experience spontaneous, often exuberant approval.

every member of our "civilized" society brings their own history with regard to the handling of strange bodies: issues relating to the socio-civilizational, to gender roles, to the small and large injuries (traumas) of their individual past and their resulting character. these are the negative aspects, the impediments which block the way. what are the positive aspects? what are the benefits?

our bodies crave connection. everyone's. there is a desire to open completely, to fuse, to give oneself to the all, to others. it may be hidden beyond recognition, through apparent hate, through autism,

8

but it remains a fundamental truth of human nature. the individual soul is longing for the universal soul, kundalini wants to return to shiva (the single life is, somehow, always reaching towards death, because it is the totality, the entropy).

every touch of another is a small step on the way there. it is beautiful, when despite the hindrances of trauma and prejudice, here in the sheltered, guided yoga room we can finally, even if briefly, overcome them. i might even truly learn to step outside of my physical isolation or restraint. the body can actually let go more of its deeply held structures when it can lean on, be held, lovingly drawn out, supported.

in the relieved sighs and deeply happy eyes of the participants, one can finds all the evidence needed to support the practice of partner stretching.
and it is yogic! it lies on the path of tantra yoga, in which the inner world opens, experience expands, is fully present, and there is space for prana.

not to be forgotten, much less devalued, here, are the sensitivities of individual participants! if i demonstrate an exercise with a student, i always ask him first if i may. this then also functions as an example for others, that they may say no if they wish. with touches on "sensitive" areas, such as the inner thigh, i make it explicit once again that they are free to skip the exercise. in one exercise, a partner places the soles of their feet on the backs of their partner's hands; here it is easy to place a blanket or put a thin pillow between them to mitigate the intimacy. in general i try not to respond to the resentments of my participants with arrogance or pity, but with love! ultimately, these objections are arising from the results of their own life history, which present themselves here to be processed and transformed.

all exercises are first demonstrated by me with a student. if three exercises or postures are to be done in sequence, usually we will show all three together. then i guide the selection of partners, mostly with the sentence: find a partner. every now and then i intervene, when the exercises require partners to be equally matched in size or strength and the students' preferences have led to an unequal pairing. in addition, after this introduction i will do the exercise as both guide and active partner, if the group is odd-numbered and needs an extra participant. it can be difficult to simultaneously manage the group, give corrections, and practice with my partner; if in doubt, i ask my current partner to briefly practice alone, and go to attend to the pairs in need of correction.

a note on the use of partner yoga exercises in children's yoga: children will all too easily express their confusion or shyness as crankiness and bad temper. thus it is very important to ensure that a loving, gentle atmosphere prevails. then partner exercises in children's yoga can be a huge success! with no need for mythical creatures, fairytales, or rewards of treats, children spontaneously express how the exercises suited them. often, they want to repeat them in the next class.

in mixed groups – in other words, boys and girls together – it's not unusual for a child to refuse to do an exercise with a particular other child as partner. here in no case should the teacher apply force. it is sufficient to make note when they show reservations, and then to ask: with whom do you think you could do that exercise? and then to ask the named student if they are willing. if on occasion a child really cannot find a partner, the teacher must take this role. but in the end everyone is always provided for, and especially for children with a tendency to be the outsider, it is a very beneficial experience to have been included in the circle of mutual touch.

4.   validated sample partner exercies, classified via five elements theory

the following examples are drawn from various classes and workshops with anando würzburger, ananda leone, daniel orlansky and jochen knau, my shiatsu teacher. in order to create a system of classification, i have grouped them via the five elements. the meridian system is well researched and described; the differentiated spheres of energy are clarified by carola beresford-cooke in *shiatsu* (see bibliography / references) or wilfried rappenecker and meike kockrick in *atlas of shiatsu* (see bibliography / references).

in choosing these exercises, i have put special value on practicality. there are a number of acrobatic exercises which completely overwhelm the average student and with certainty will lead to dissatisfaction. the touch of others, in its physical reality, is in itself already a challenge; if in addition, the level of challenge of the exercises is too high, this is asking for frustration and resentment. likewise, some wonderful exercises are simply too intimate to pursue in an ordinary yoga group. physical contacts must be pursued in stages, and whether through a yoga belt, or on the inner side of the thighs, or to the face, can only via delicacy and compassion be enjoyed.

within an exercise, several meridians are usually activated; listing each with specific "organs" and elemental phases of transformation is to be understood as merely a general guide. the featured partner exercises can also be used individually as invited by the overall structure of the class. for example, in a class focused on the mobilization and invigoration of the parts of the shoulder, it might make sense to include a partner exercise integrating back and shoulder massage. i have found, however, that a series of several partner exercises can improve and refine the attention of the partners. i have had much success with a sequence of three partner exercises per class. accordingly, my presentation is divided into sequences of three. in the main, one partner leads the other through all three exercises, before then changing roles.

the following table contains one photo per exercise. the notes are brief; of course, each exercise in turn contains a whole universe of meanings and possibilities, both for variation and for potential mistakes! those with little experience with bodywork will do best to remain on the more superficial level of opening and movement, finding their own stable understanding; and at this stage will feel the lack of more guidance. but you have to start somewhere, and i have a learned a great deal through common practice with my students.

what is shown in the photos will not be reiterated in the text. the duration of one exercise, once all postures are taken in and both partners involve themselves, should, as a rule, take about a minute. less time would be insufficient to focus concentration, and with much longer, they could again under some circumstances go astray.

for each elemental phase, there are two proposed exercises, with the exception of water, where there are four. the "water organs" of bladder and kidney are of particularly great importance, as the bladder governs the back and the kidney reflects fundamental life force.

(note in german: as most of the pictured models are female, i have chosen to balance this by writing the descriptions in the male gender. in the english translation, this has been addressed by writing in gender-neutral terms.)

class		
elemental phase organ **focus** energetic quality **overview**		
1 **metal** lung / large intestine **communication** vitality / anxiety **lung meridian** lungen- meridian 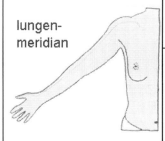 **large intestine meridian** dick- darm- meridian 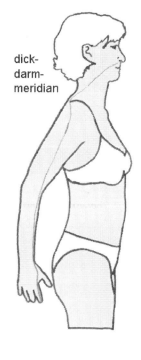	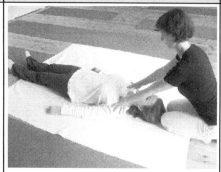	**lung 1** the lung meridian begins arouond 2 cm. under the collarbones. the „lung 1" point lies around the middle of the palpable section of each clavicle bone. the two outstretched thumbs of the active partner, as a rule, „fall" „by themselves" into this very important energetic point. 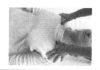
	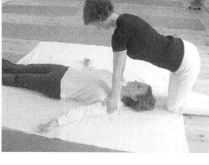	**shoulder–catwalk** first the body weight is brought to bear on the shoulders; then the active partner begins to gently shift the weight from side to side.
	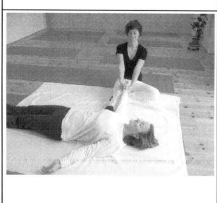	**arm extension** one of the practitioner's feet – ideally, wearing socks – is placed in the armpit area of the supine partner. the hand is held gently but firmly at the wrist. by leaning back, the arm is gently drawn out of the socket. the difficult task of the passive partner: let go! focus: to bring the six arm meridians to the fore.

2

metal

lung / large intestine

communication

vitality / anxiety

lung meridian

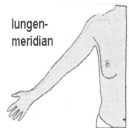

lungen-
meridian

**large intestine
meridian**

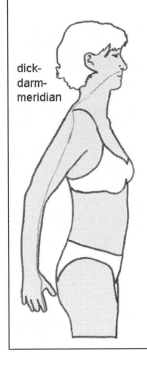

dick-
darm-
meridian

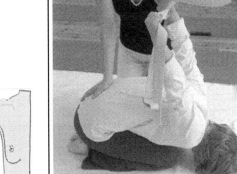

the rabbit

the secure and balanced pressure of the resting hand on the lower back is important here. the receiving partner holds a strap between the hands – even if it is easy to bring the hands together, the belt makes this posture softer and gentler. the active partner gently moves the arms in the direction of the head. the partners must communicate about a comfortable degree of stretch! a cushion under the forehead can be lovely.

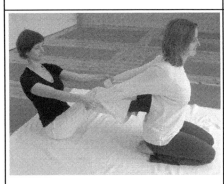

back-walk

walk the feet up and down along the outsides of the spine, stopping from time to time... pressing toes under the shoulder blade, resting a heel lightly on the kidney...

the active partner can also work leaning against a wall, to save work in the core muscles.

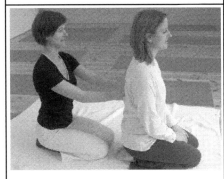

smooth out the back

slowly and with deep attention, stroke the back from top to bottom three times. focus: let the contents of the mind release out into the earth.

3

earth

stomach / spleen

grounding

compassion / reticence

stomach meridian

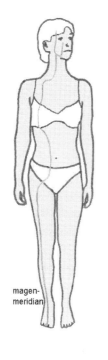

magen-
meridian

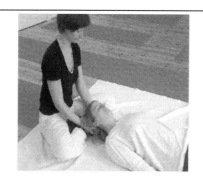

losing one's head

the partner's head is securely held in both hands, and lightly and irregularly moved here and there, up and down, back and forth. task of the receiver: to relax the neck muscles so completely that the head can be simultaneously as heavy as lead, as light as a feather.

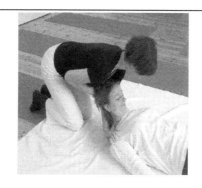

the chin kisses the chest

one hand holds the head from below. the other reaches through, under the first arm to the opposite shoulder, and with the palm downward, holds the tip of the shoulder with the fingertips. the partners synchronize breath. on the exhale, lower the reclining partner's head forward until resistance is felt. on the inhale, return the head to the starting position. change sides.

wipe away your cares

with your thumbs, stroke the forehead several times at varying heights from the center outwards towards the temples. with the disappearance of the outward wrinkles, all the worries within melt away!

4

earth

stomach / spleen

grounding

compassion / reticence

spleen meridian

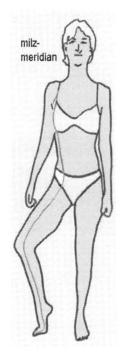

milz-
meridian

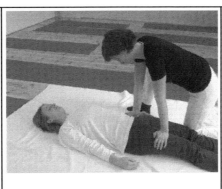

making space in the belly

one hand rests a portion of the body weight on the hip joint of one side. the other hand very slowly works its way up and down the opposite thigh. the fingers should always point outward! the back and forth-leaning movement of the active partner should emanate directly from your center, the hara-point under the navel.

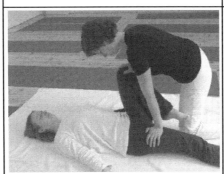

press out the belly

the raised knee is moved gently against the resistance in the hip. many experience unpleasant pressure in the lymph nodes of the groin area here; so work cautiously, begin very gently, keep asking. the other hand firmly stabilizes the opposite thigh. the flexed leg can move back and forth a few times or even be rotated in outward circles.

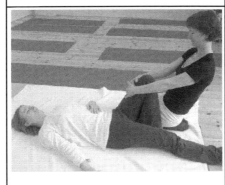

release the lower back

hold the engaged leg with both hands securely below the knee and pull it towards you. the practitioner may also stabilize the engaged foot on the floor with their knees. move the leg back and forth several times.

5

fire

heart / small intestine

activity

joy / melancholy

heart meridian

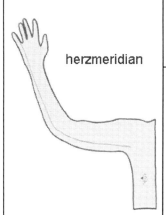

herzmeridian

small intestine meridian

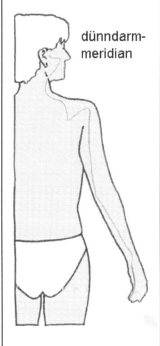

dünndarm-meridian

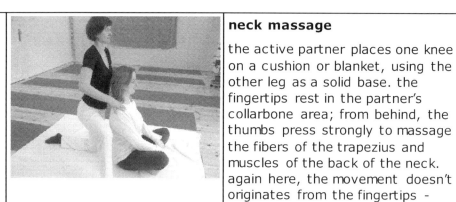

neck massage

the active partner places one knee on a cushion or blanket, using the other leg as a solid base. the fingertips rest in the partner's collarbone area; from behind, the thumbs press strongly to massage the fibers of the trapezius and muscles of the back of the neck. again here, the movement doesn't originates from the fingertips - rather the entire body participates!

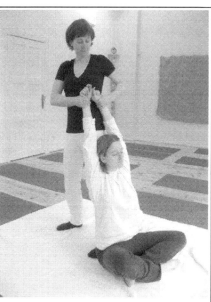

opening by leaning!

with the receiving partner seated cross-legged, place one foot with the outer edge behind the buttocks. hold the wrists firmly and lay them on the side (avoid contact with the breast region!) of your upper body. then, by bending the back leg, shift the weight, and stretch the partner's upper body lengthwise, gently but firmly. avoid pulling the partner through your own shoulder and arm strength – this is strenuous, and the exertion transmits itself to your partner. when the exercise is properly arranged, it will happen easily.

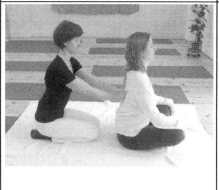

smooth out the back

slowly and with deep attention, stroke the back from top to bottom three times. focus: let the contents of the mind release out into the earth.

6
fire

heart / small intestine

activity

joy /melancholy

heart meridian

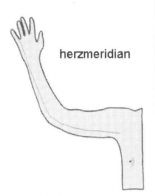

herzmeridian

small intestine meridian

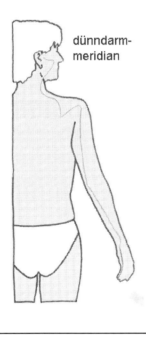

dünndarm-meridian

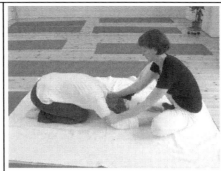

wring out the arms

squeeze out the tissues of the arms as if you were wringing out a sponge. in particular, the tissues of the lymph system can only renew themselves via this outer pressure, and are very grateful for such massage.

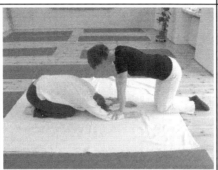

arm walkabout

with smooth, even pressure, press out the forearms and hands, using the balls of your hands. exercise caution in the areas of the joints. don't forget the backs of the hands and the fingers!

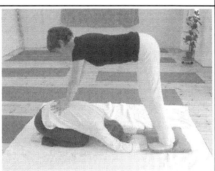

push the back long

lay the receiving partner's hands on a cushion, and then stand on them with both feet. place your own hands to the lower back and lean your full weight into them. the hands fixed to the floor give an unusual feeling of being at your partner's mercy.

the kidneys enjoy this warm pressure – a happy side effect of this stretching of the back!

7

water

bladder / kidney

identity

courage / fear

bladder meridian

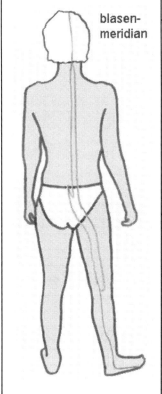

blasen-meridian

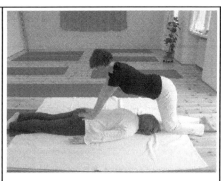

leaning on the iliac crest

let all your available weight flow through your hands. remain still.

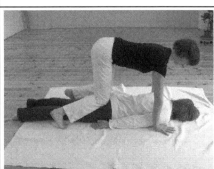

kneel on the bottom

the receiving partner lies on their belly – first tell them you will be stepping across them. then place your hands next to their shoulders, and slowly let the knees sink into the buttocks. for the most part, your can give your full weight; but it's best to communicate about this beforehand.

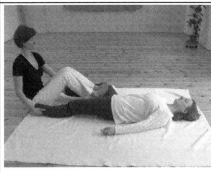

inner thigh foot massage

very pleasant, but very delicate! advise your partner that their sensitivies may be offended, but let them know that this is an extremely effective massage for muscles, vessels and meridians which rarely receive such treatment. i would not offer this in all groups. this exercise comes out of traditional thai massage.

8

water

bladder / kidney

identity

courage / fear

kidney meridian (beginning)

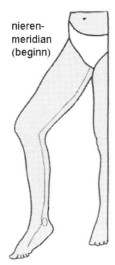

nieren-meridian (beginn)

kidney meridian (ending)

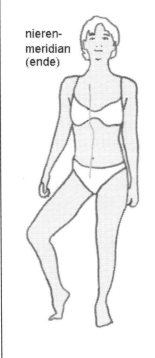

nieren-meridian (ende)

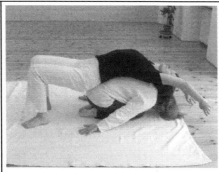

lying backwards over the back

a deep backbend, especially if the partner on top extends their arms back. it's important to position the pelvis as low as possible, so that the backbend can travel over the highest point of the partner underneath. a nice experience for the bottom partner as well, who is „pressed out"!

carry your partner

first stand facing each other, hold hands, then raise the arms and turn to come back to back. the bottom partner bends the knees enough to bring their buttocks under those of their partner. then they stretch their arms overhead as much as possible, and bend forward, stretching their partner out over their back. a deep stretch! do not add any additional swinging or movements. insofar as possible, partners should be of equivalent weight. with experience, one can easily work with a larger partner.

the see-saw straddle

if the legs of the partners are of unequal length or more or less wide in the straddle, the feet can also be brought to the lower legs of the opposing partner. bend forward and hold for several breaths, and then bend backwards and again hold. a circular movement is also possible here: as if we're stirring a enormous pot of soup with a huge spoon!

9

water

bladder / kidney

identity

courage / fear

bladder meridian

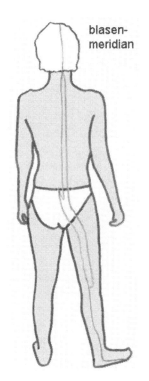

blasen-
meridian

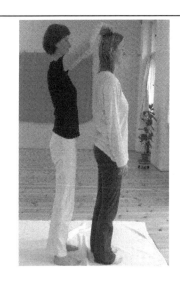

the kidney rainshower

the fingertips rain gently on the head. the receiving partner feels the water flow downward from their hair over their shoulders, throughout the entire body... the light fingertips gradually make their way down both sides of the arms all the way out to the hands.

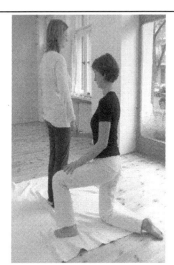

shaking hands

the active partner kneels on a blanket or cushion next to the receiving partner, and grasps one of their thumbs firmly with a hand. with a gentle pull, they begin to swing the arm side to side. this is intended to provide a vibration with which the entire body can resonate. the standing partner's task is to become so soft in the muscles and joints as to allow this vibration to be perceptibly spread throughout the entire body. if there is enough time, it is worth working through all the fingers.

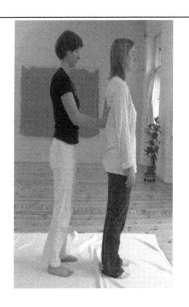

smooth out the body

with your whole body fully engaged from the crown of the head to the soles of your feet, and with both hands, smooth out down the sides of your partner's spine and legs.

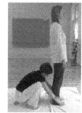

after the third time, let the hands rest quietly on the tops of the feet, thus connecting the feet with the earth.

10

water

bladder / kidney

identity

courage / fear

kidney meridan (beginning)

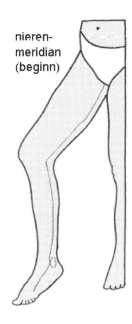

nieren-
meridian
(beginn)

kidney meridian (ending)

nieren-
meridian
(ende)

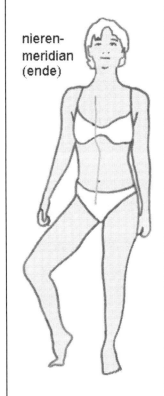

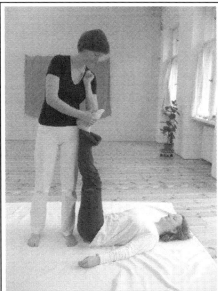

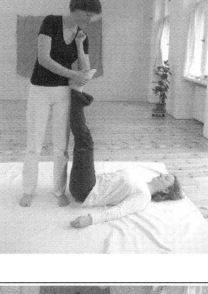

kidney 1

the kidney meridian originates in the center ball of the sole of the foot. deep pressure here activates the quality of vitality. in addition, the elbow has a particular ability to transmit energy. place the feet at your side and with each elbow, work on both feet; thus between sides, turn your opposite side to your receiving partner.

carry the legs by the big toe

hold both big toes firmly and very slowly lower the legs to the floor. most partners will try to „help" by holding on in the legs. then must you protest: „let go!"

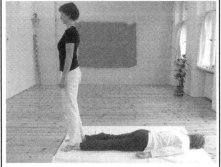

walking in a stranger's shoes

first: „put on your socks, if you wish". then very consciously and deliberately „walk" on the soles, vigorously massaging the feet. end with tiny gentle steps on the toes.

11
secondary fire

pericardium / triple warmer

activity

joy / melancholy

pericardium meridian

pericard-meridian

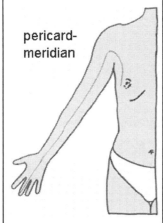

triple warmer meridian

Dreifacher
Wärmer
Meridian

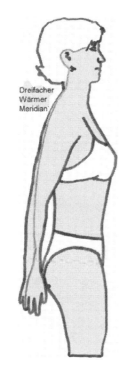

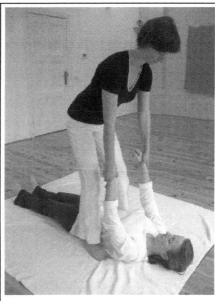

lift the arms out of the shoulders

... very gently! this is only a very subtle movement in the shoulders. the receiving partner again has the most difficult task: from inside, to truly surrender!

we work again with leaning and body weight here. the shifting back and forth of the body moves the arm – the muscles of the arm and shoulder are not engaged!

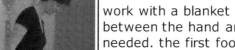

massaging the arm with the foot

work with a blanket or cushion between the hand and foot as needed. the first foot grounds the hand; the other foot walks back and forth along the inside edge of the forearm. the active partner should maintain consistent, even pressure! it is an interesting experience of foot energy for the receiving partner. many emotions connected

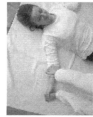

with daily pleasures and discomforts reside in the muscles and joints of the arms!

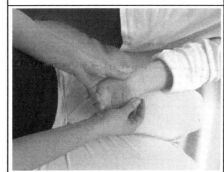

hand massage

interlace your pinky fingers next to the pinky finger and thumb. rest the hands on your own thigh or the floor. the thumbs massage the wrist and palm, while the fingertips work from behind into the back of the hand.

12
secondary fire

pericardium / triple warmer

activity

joy / melancholy

pericardium meridian

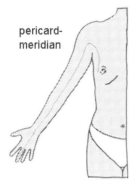

pericard-meridian

triple warmer meridian

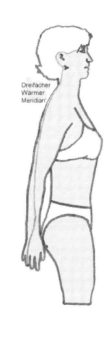

Dreifacher Wärmer Meridian

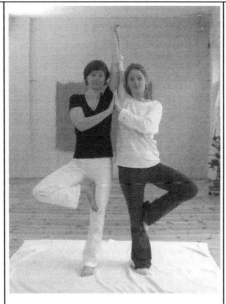

twinned tree 1

two on one leg is far easier than one alone!

so that it isn't too easy, stay on the same leg and shift into the second form (see below).

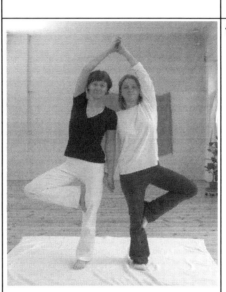

twinned tree 2

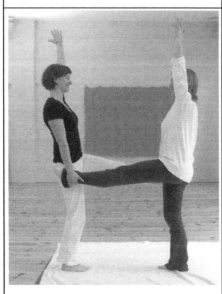

the big "h"

it's not as easy as it looks!

13

wood

gallblader / liver

growth

enthusiasm / anger

gallblader meridian

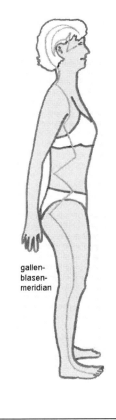

gallen-
blasen-
meridian

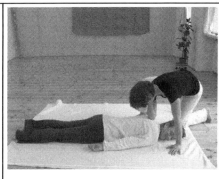

the back point

in one point along the gallblader meridian in the upper back, the story of the entire back manifests. the elbow will fit naturally into this point! the direction of pressure should point inward toward the body, so somewhat slanted, as shown in the picture, where the elbow is nearly sliding off.

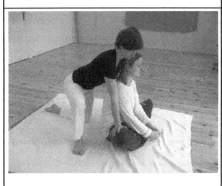

butterfly

a support for this groin stretch. do not bounce, but rather remain still. support the forward bend in the back by leaning against it, deepen the legs toward the earth through gentle pressure. fingertips face back toward the active partner.

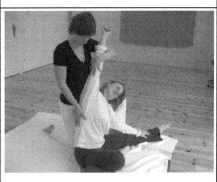

side bend

support your partner so they do not need to use their own energy to stay upright. this gives them more buoyancy for the side bend. give the arm direction and through touch, help the stretching side to „open".

14

wood

gallblader / liver

growth

enthusiasm / anger

liver meridian

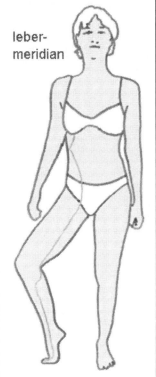

leber-
meridian

---

standing twist

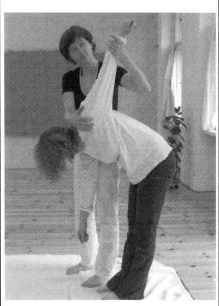

support the lower shoulder with your hips while stabilizing the upper shoulder with your entire hand and drawing it upward. naturally, go only so far as your partner can tolerate. ask! the ideal time, when the body is soft: in summer, not too early in the day, after vigorous practice.

---

beat out the back in a forward bend

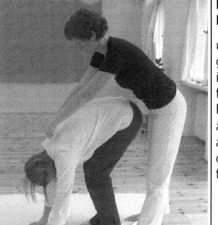

use a hollow hand and the fingers gently tucked in, so that the contact is with the second phalanx of the finger bones. like the clapper of a bell, the hands should land in an alternating pattern, the wrists soft and relaxed. from the shoulders over the backs of the legs to the feet, three times.

---

the chi machine

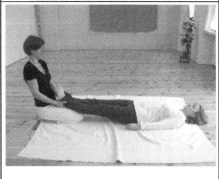

... one can also buy one. a device which rhythmically oscillates the legs back and forth. immensely enjoyable! apply a gentle pull (this the machine can't do!) when the passive partner gives themselves completely over, the head will nod along. this should allow the body to return to its proper frequency.

5.   experiential report of reintegration into the astanga sadhana of swami gitananda

in accordance with my tradition (following swami gitananda giri), my classes have an integrated eight-step structure:

1.   class begins with the **arrival** into practice, mostly through reclined floor work, a few openings and stretches **(mudra).**

2.   this is followed by a few words from the teacher regarding motivation, **attitude / intention**, linking the yoga practice together with the spiritual cosmos **(puja).**

3.   a short verse or tone sung together connects the individual with the whole in the **vibration** of the present moment **(mantra).**

4.   movement then begins with a **(kriya),** meaning, a **sequence of movements** that is guided by the breath which mobilizes the body and breath.

5.   now come the **yoga postures (asanas),** which usually form the focus of the class. at the beginning, preparatory poses and leading poses, care being taken that all directions of stretching and turning, as well as inversions, receive attention. as a rule, the peak of the class occurs here in with a well-prepared, level-appropriate challenging pose.

afterward we arrive at the practice of the above-described **meridian-opening exercises**. body and mind are ideally supple; the peak of the class has been achieved; the partner exercises offer the opportunity to again emerge from individual-ness and share and enjoy the rediscovered openness **with a partner.**

6.   at the end, all again find their own comfortable seat, and together the group performs practices linking **breath and life force (pranayama).**

7.   usually returning to reclining on the floor, this is followed by **relaxation**, bringing quiet to the body and mind to greatest possible extent **(nispanda).**

8.   finally, sitting in meditation, concentration and contemplation have hopefully reached their peak; the babble of the mind, for at least a moment, departs, and there is stillness. **(dharana/dhyana)** at the very closing, we again sing the mantra *om*, and perhaps a further sanskrit verse. then we bow and greet the universe, our teacher, the group and ourselves and the earth, on which we live.

6. summary

partner exercises are well suited to the intensive observation of individual yoga asanas. they are used regularly for this reason, as well as for support in difficult poses.

in this work i wanted to share my experience that it is well worth making meridian-opening partner exercises a consistent part of group yoga practice over a longer timespan.

such partner exercises provide a deeper realm of experience with a number of advantages:

intensification	one's own body perception is deepened through exchange
concentration	attending to your partner's inner experience prevents distraction
communication	making contact and practicing with others
mirroring	one's own movements can be observed in a stranger's body
opening	expansion and sharing of personal vitality / life energy
tantra	the sensory experience of the world is enriched by new spaces
yoga	the individual soul progresses toward the universal soul
support	the other supports „daring" postures and poses
healing	the dismantling of hurts connected with physical contact
variation	a new perspective on old familar parts of the body

a class composed solely of partner exercises would, i think, be problematic, for yoga is and remains first a practice of self-awareness.

integrated into a structured class, however, meridian-opening exercises offer my students and me an inspired source of enrichment.

thomas propp, summer 2009

i welcome suggestions and corrections: thomas@yogalila.de

7. bibliography / references

leone, ananda and the group in the yoga teacher training in the berlin academy for yoga, script and protocol of the trainings in the timeframe from 23.09.2005 to 23.04.2009

alex, irina and **schmidt, valentin;** „partner yoga", article in *yoga aktuell* number 52, october/november 2008

beresford-cooke, carola; *shiatsu, fundamentals and practice,* munich 2001 (urban & fischer verlag)

eliade, mircea; *yoga – immortality and freedom*, frankfurt 1985 (suhrkamp taschenbuch 1127)

knau, jochen; *handbook of zen-shiatsu*, berlin 2002, unpublished manuscript (self-published)

masunaga, shitsuto / ohashi, wataru; *the big book of healing through shiatsu,* bern-münchen-wien 2000 (o. w. barth-verlag)

mayer, heike and **iding, doris;** *partner yoga*, petersberg 2003 (vianova verlag)

ohashi, wataru; *shiatsu, the japanese finger pressure therapy,* freiburg 1977 (bauer verlag)

rappenecker, wilfried; *shiatsu for beginners*, munich 2001 (wilhelm goldmann verlag)

patanjali; *the yoga sutras, in translation by sri ram*, berlin 2006 (theseus)

rappenecker, wilfried / kockrick, meike; *atlas of shiatsu, the meridians of zen-shiatsu*, munich 2007 (urban & fischer verlag)

würzburger, anando / ruhnke, amiyo; *body-wisdom*, munich 1997 (knaur verlag)

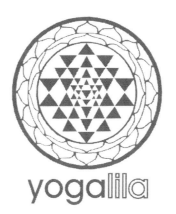

yogalila

thomas propp
thomas@yogalila.de
english translation by julie blumenthal
copyright: © 2012 thomas propp

Made in the USA
San Bernardino, CA
03 January 2018